70 Top Gree... Re...

Smoothie Detox For A Sexy ...atnful You

By: Samantha Michaels

TABLE OF CONTENTS

Samantha Michaels

PUBLISHERS NOTES

Disclaimer

This publication is intended to provide helpful and informative material. It is not intended to diagnose, treat, cure, or prevent any health problem or condition, nor is intended to replace the advice of a physician. No action should be taken solely on the contents of this book. Always consult your physician or qualified health-care professional on any matters regarding your health and before adopting any suggestions in this book or drawing inferences from it.

The author and publisher specifically disclaim all responsibility for any liability, loss or risk, personal or otherwise, which is incurred as a consequence, directly or indirectly, from the use or application of any contents of this book.

Any and all product names referenced within this book are the trademarks of their respective owners. None of these owners have sponsored, authorized, endorsed, or approved this book.

Always read all information provided by the manufacturers' product labels before using their products. The author and publisher are not responsible for claims made by manufacturers.

© 2013

Manufactured in the United States of America

DEDICATION

This book is dedicated to my father Jim who inspired me to follow my dreams.

Chapter 1- The History of the Green Smoothie

Green smoothies are popular among those seeking a healthy lifestyle. Touted as the ideal healthy snack and even a nutritious meal replacement, green smoothies are found on many café and street vendor menus. Their rise to fame is attributed to the increased popularity of the health and weight-loss shakes that have swept the nation. Consumers searching for a more nutrient-rich, dairy-free or low-fat option, helped to bring the green smoothie to the forefront.

With fresh, organic produce readily available, more people are embracing the green trend, whipping up green smoothies at home. Believers in the green smoothie are reaping the health benefits of these fresh satisfying concoctions that are void of preservatives and additives. The thing is that the green smoothie is anything but a new sensation.

Traditionally, a smoothie is a blended drink, made of fruit, milk and yogurt. Some recipes call for fruit juices to avoid dairy products. Over the years this blend has become more specialized and now features many variations. It is important to point out that smoothies are not milkshakes. Smoothies use whole fruits and vegetables, whereas milkshake tends to add flavor-enhancers and sweeteners to milk. Smoothies are typically thicker than a milkshake too. Smoothies aren't only made from the juice of fruits and vegetables either; hence their nutritional value does differ to that of juicing foods. This is an important distinction, as often juicing is done to enjoy the flavor of certain fruits and vegetables. When it comes to green smoothies, the vegetables are not always selected for their taste. Their essential vitamins, minerals and dietary fiber far outweigh any flavor they add to a drink.

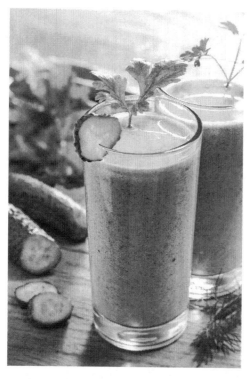

Who coined the name "smoothie" is not really known. The oldest patent associated with the title belongs to Stephen Kuhnau, who established the 1970s Smoothie King franchise. But historically, the concept of a smoothie traces back further. The traditional drink of India, known as a "lasse" bears a remarkable resemblance to a smoothie. It is a blend of yoghurt, fruit, honey and spices, and was around before the birth of Christ. In Brazil, drinks made of fruit purée blended with yogurt also feature in antiquity. Oddly enough, thick, creamy drinks containing avocado and other fruits are traditional fare in Vietnam, the Philippines and Indonesia. The 1920s and 1930s saw entrepreneurs promote these foreign elixirs in health stores across the West Coast of America.

As technology developed, so did the smoothie. The 1920s saw the birth of household appliances. Homes soon filled with machines that made life easier. One of these highly valued kitchen accessories was the blender. The 1933 "Miracle Mixer" is accredited for its efforts in establishing the "smoothie" as a household name. It, along with the improved models released well into the 1940s, all featured smoothie recipes in their accompanying cookbooks. As the technology developed machines capable of combining ingredients into smooth, thick liquids, the smoothie became more popular.

By the 1960s, typical smoothie blends saw fruits, fruit juices or milk being whipped together in tasty treats. The 1970s embraced the trend of using frozen yoghurt in smoothies. The 1980s added supplements; experimenting with protein and vitamin powders. Yet it was the 1990s that heralded a new smoothie renaissance, giving birth to a multi-billion dollar industry across the Western World: but what of the green smoothie?

Victoria Boutenko introduced the green smoothie at a time when smoothies become more popular than ever. Tired of constant, niggling health issues, Boutenko decided to try the all-natural, raw foods diet. In the 1990s, she subjected herself, and her family, to a decade long diet that strictly had them eating meals rich in green, leafy produce.

Strangely enough, her research compared the Standard American Diet (SAD) with the typical diet of our closest living relative, the chimpanzee. She found that chimps ate a diet of at least forty percent leafy greens and fifty percent fruit. The highly promoted raw-food diet encouraged extremely high amounts of fruit, and recommended only ten percent of leafy greens per day. Boutenko began exploring the benefits of increasing the greens in their diet. Based on her research, and her own family's experiences, Boutenko found green smoothies to be the greatest health choice.

Victoria Boutenko recommended that the average person needed to consume at least four servings of green leaves and up to four pounds of fresh fruit each day. Although most people could stomach the fruit, munching down large servings of salad leaves became a chore. Further research also revealed that the full nutritional value of green leafy vegetables was only fully gained when the cell walls of the leaves were chewed, or cut.

The smaller the leaves were shredded, the better they were for the digestive system. This information led to the development of the green smoothie. By using a high-grade blender, green leafy matter such as spinach, was easily chopped into a smooth substance that mixed very well with fruit and a little water. The generous serving of fruits masked any bitter taste of a variety of fresh leaves, creating a drink that was highly nutritional; and so the green smoothie revolution begun.

Today, many people are experiencing the benefits of drinking green smoothies. There are hundreds of recipe books and websites that are dedicated to creating varied and tasty versions of this health tonic. Green smoothies promise to offer a low-calorie, highly nutritional boost to the diet. They contain essential vitamins and trace elements that can only be sourced from the hero of the drink, the green leafy vegetables. Green smoothies are said to help with digestive issues, but have also been recommended to ease rheumatoid arthritis and many allergies and other health concerns. Today, the green smoothie continues to evolve as new blends and products are explored.

CHAPTER 2- THE BENEFITS OF GREEN SMOOTHIES

A lot of health fanatics love to drink smoothies. Some people make a green smoothie for breakfast while other people drink a smoothie before they lift weights. Smoothies have gained in popularity as they are easy to make and can be made on the go. Beyond that, most health conscious people would agree that a green smoothie is a perfect snack or meal anytime of the day. For these reasons, green smoothies have exploded in popularity. Here are ten benefits of green smoothies.

Most people do not drink enough water, and a smoothie is an excellent way to get the required eight glasses of water per day. In fact, a smoothie drinker who does not get enough water can add water to their smoothie. This is a good way to get hydrated without even thinking about it. Though overlooked, smoothies help with a person's hydration.

The great thing about green smoothies is; they are easy to make. A person who has no skills in the kitchen can make a green smoothie with ease. As far as supplies, all one needs is a blender and a large pitcher if they want to store the excess amounts. Anyone can make a smoothie within a couple of minutes. Most people already have of the necessary equipment needed to make a smoothie.

Anyone with digestion problems should consider making green smoothies. With a smoothie, the body does not need to work hard to break down the food to get the nutrients. Not only that, anyone with indigestion should consider making a smoothie as they are a light snack that is still filling. While a person can eat raw fruits and vegetables for the same effect, most people prefer a smoothie as it goes down easier than raw food. A lot of people have discovered that they do not need expensive medication or therapy once they switch to drinking smoothies.

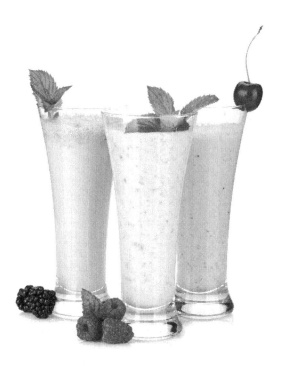

The biggest reason most people drink a green smoothie is for their health. Smoothies are one of the healthiest snacks or meal a person can eat. A dieter can get their required fruits and vegetables with a smoothie without thinking. When making a smoothie in the morning, a dieter can add a lot of fruits and vegetables with ease, making the drink taste terrific while also being healthy. Smoothies are perfect for children as it is easy to get children to eat their vegetables without forcing them.

The cost to make a smoothie is low as it is easy to buy fruits and vegetables in bulk. When buying supplies for a smoothie, it is easy to put excess supplies in the refrigerator and freezer. Many people who make smoothies have it down to an art and are able to make a smoothie cheaply. A smoothie drinker does not need to buy the expensive and best looking fruits; when making smoothies one can buy the older fruits and vegetables as it does not matter as one will put all of their fruits in a blender. Simply put; smoothies are a cheap and healthy alternative to most meals.

A lot of gym goers love smoothies. Most people love to have a pre or post workout meal. As most gym goers are health conscious, a smoothie is a perfect option to keep the body healthy and hydrated. Since there is no set smoothie recipe, exercisers of all lifestyles love to make a post workout smoothie. Anyone looking to bulk up can easily add protein powder while someone looking to lose weight can have a low-calorie smoothie. In the end, a serious exerciser should have a green smoothie before or after their workout. A smoothie is a perfect meal no matter what goal the exerciser has.

As mentioned, green smoothies offer an excellent source of energy. Unfortunately, a lot of people rely on coffee and donuts for their energy in the morning. When one has coffee and donuts, they will experience a spike in energy followed by a crash. Since a smoothie has a lot of fruits and vegetables, the drinker of a smoothie will have a lot of energy throughout the day without losing energy. Fruits and vegetables have a lot of fiber and vitamins, which help an individual stay energetic throughout the day.

Most people, inevitably, get sick during the holidays. People get sick because they are in close-quarters with other people and end up picking up other people's germs. While it is difficult to prevent this; a healthy eater will not get sick as often. When drinking a smoothing every morning, the body will have a stronger immune system. With a strong immune system, it is easier to fight off the flu or the common cold. When a person must have avoid getting sick, he or she should have a smoothie a day to make sure that they have a healthy immune system.

Cooking is fun for most people. Unfortunately, most people hate to clean up dirty dishes and pots and pans. When making a smoothie, one does not need to worry about cleaning up a large mess. Other than washing off the knife and blender, there is almost nothing to clean when making a smoothie. When one can rinse out their blender, they will only be left with, at most, a five-minute cleaning job. Anyone at work can clean their blender with ease as it only takes a few minutes to clean it in the sink. In the end, anyone who hates cleaning should consider buying a blender and making smoothies.

Smoothies are not a fad. There are plenty of health benefits to drinking a smoothie. Many people enjoy a green smoothie as they can tweak the recipe exactly as they want. While people enjoy the health benefits, a lot of working professionals also love the convenience of a green smoothie. One can make a smoothie without making a mess. A lot of people have discovered that when they make smoothies, not only will they save money they will be a lot healthier.

CHAPTER 3- HOW TO MAKE GREEN SMOOTHIES

You'll need a blender and some spinach, a banana, some strawberries and your choice of soy milk or almond milk. Blend all these ingredients together adding each one slowly. Once you see that it's all blended together you can enjoy your green smoothie. This is one way recipe for a green smoothie and you will learn that there are lots of other recipes.

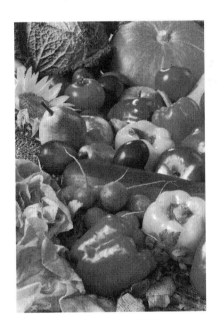

You can get two bananas, a half of a cup of your choice of a pineapple, apple or a peach plus you'll need sixteen ounces of water and one and a half cups of kale or spinach. Blend these ingredients together until it's smooth. If you want the smoothie as smooth as possible, just blend for a longer amount of time to get it extra smooth.

Another tip is that if you want your smoothie colder, take all the ingredients and freeze them over night or you can add some ice cubes in the blender too. The amount of time spent in blending all these ingredients together will depend on the blender you are using and the way you prefer your smoothie. Don't be afraid to blend everything for a longer period if you like your smoothies smooth. There is not right amount of time or no wrong amount of time to keep your ingredients blending because it's all your choice.

You can add anything you'd like to the ingredients to make a smoothie so don't be afraid to add and or take out some ingredients. Once you get to making smoothies, you'll know just how you like yours and which ingredients that you prefer. There are recipe books that can help tell you which ingredients to add and which to leave out. You can make different green smoothies every day if you prefer to change it up but if you do that, remember to write the ingredients down if you want to make that same one again.

The smoothies are not only tasty but they are nutritious for you. You'll be getting a smoothie that you love with vegetables and fruits recommended for you. If you aren't eating your fruits or vegetables but are drinking them, it's the very same thing plus you are getting your daily allowance. When you add the fruit to these smoothies the taste of the fruit is what you will taste.

As you continue to drink these green smoothies you'll see that you body won't need or crave the junk foods or the sweets, now you'll be balancing out your diet with the fruits and vegetables and you are going to see a weight loss as well. If a person cannot eat raw vegetables, drinking a green smoothie is the best way for them to have all of their vitamins and nutrients that a person needs daily.

The green smoothies are going to give you energy that you need so you can start a workout program if you aren't on one. You'll see that you are going to spend less time in the kitchen as the green smoothies are very easy to make. Add whatever you want to the smoothie and drink up. If you like the smoothie because it tastes good, keep drinking it. You don't have to know that this is all healthy for you. You can use frozen or fresh fruits when you make your green smoothies as either way it will be fine.

As healthy as a green smoothie is, you'll want to make it healthier by getting the daily exercise you will need and the rest that is recommended, plus you're still going to need to drink lots of water. Trying for a stress free life is what is going to make us happy and healthier. Learn how to take better care yourself too. Watch your alcohol intake if you are choosing to become healthy and keep on drinking these green smoothies for your fruit and vegetable intake.

You can enjoy a green smoothie any time of the day either will a meal or for a snack. There are juice bars that offer lots of different green smoothies. Order one with all the veggies and fruits that you love even when you're away from home.

When you first start making green smoothies try to put more fruits in the juicer and make it sweet to start with. As you get used to drinking the smoothie, start to add more and more vegetables to it so that you will gradually get used to the taste.

Green smoothies are great for the parents of the children that refuse to eat their vegetables and don't care much for fruit. Give them a green smoothie and they'll be sure to drink it and get their quantity of the vegetables their bodies need. Let them help you make it too, that's all the fun leading up to this tasty drink. Soon they'll be making their own and making yours as well. They can have this drink as a snack or with any of their meals. Either way, they are getting their daily vegetables and fruits.

You can blend anything healthy into a green smoothie, peanut butter, raisins, some yogurt if you'd like. Anything that you have on hand and is good for you, try it. Add either water or ice cubes or both to the mix. If the green smoothie comes out as good as you expected just write down all the ingredients that you used for the next time when you want that very same taste.

CHAPTER 4- 14 GREAT BREAKFAST GREEN SMOOTHIE RECIPES

We have all heard the tip about breakfast being the most important meal of the day. Are you looking for a nice cool refreshing drink to start your day off right? Start the day with a wonderful burst of green from a refreshing and energy-boosting smoothie blend. You will love these cool tasty smoothies and your body will love to wake up to them as well. These satisfying green treats are super healthy for you. Smoothies are easy to digest and get nutrients flowing throughout your body quickly for an early morning start. There are a variety of green smoothie recipes. Choose the one that suits your taste buds.

Do not limit these great recipes to breakfast time. Adopt them as your new daily vitamin drink. Serve them for some tasty holiday party flair. Serve them for any special occasion, or for a causal fun treat? Once you master these recipes, your guests are sure to be impressed by how sweet and flavorful these healthy smoothies can be.

The key to making a healthy green smoothie is to make your smoothie with about forty percent green vegetables. The blend of fruits and veggies will boost your body with a refreshing burst of nutrients and energy.

Blending Tips:

The consistency of your smoothie will depend upon the type of blender that you are using. If you are using a strong, high quality blender, you will be able to blend up almost anything in your smoothie. If you are using a below average blender, you might end up with a chunky smoothie. Therefore, please consider that fact that you might need some of your ingredients to be crushed or ground up before adding them into the blender. You might also need to peel the skins off some of the ingredients.

No matter what type of blender you have, it is always a good idea to cut up the fruits and veggies before adding them to the blender. There is no need to dice or slice. Just get things cut into big chunks as opposed to adding large, whole fruits and veggies.

You can gradually add things into the blender as you make your smoothie, or you can layer the ingredients. Here is the best order to add and layer your ingredients: liquids, dry and powder ingredients, leafy ingredients, fruit and veggies pieces, and ice cubes on the top. Putting the heavier ingredients on top will help to weigh down leafy ingredients into the blender blades. Then of course, you blend it until it is smooth.

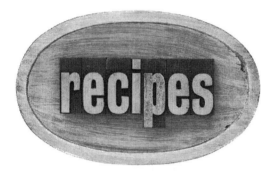

Here are fourteen amazing green smoothie blends for you to enjoy.

Mean Green Detox Machine
1/2 cup orange juice
2 teaspoons ginger
2 cups kale
1/2 cup cilantro
1 lime (remove the seeds, keep the peel)
1 green apple
1 banana (frozen, chopped)

Directions
Blend all the ingredients.

Green Leafy Smoothie
1/2 cup apple juice
2 cups mixed greens
1 cup spinach
1 lemon (remove the seeds, keep the peel)
1 pear
1 banana (frozen, chopped)
Directions
Blend all the ingredients.

Green Avocado Smoothie
3/4 cup coconut water
1/2 cup kale
1/2 cup spinach
1/2 cup avocado
2 cups seedless grapes
1 pear
4 - 5 ice cubes
Directions
Blend all the ingredients.

Green Carrot Smoothie
1/2 cup water
1/2 cup skim milk
1/2 tsp. cinnamon
1/8 cup old-fashioned rolled oats
1/2 cup spinach
2 small carrots or 1 large carrot (with green tops)
1 banana (frozen, chopped)
4 - 5 ice cubes
Directions
Blend all the ingredients.

Green Melon Smoothie

1/2 cup water

3 tbsp. honey

1 lime wedge (remove the seeds, keep the peel)

1 cup kale

1/2 cup cantaloupe

1/2 cup honeydew

4 - 5 ice cubes Directions

Blend all the ingredients.

Refreshing Cucumber Delight

1/2 cup water

4 tbsp. honey

2 cups kale

1 lime wedge (remove the seeds, keep the peel)

2 cucumbers (remove seeds and peel)

4 - 5 ice cubes

Directions

Blend all the ingredients.

Berry Green Smoothie

1/2 cup apple juice

1 cup spinach

2 cups mixed berries

1 banana (frozen, chopped)

4 - 5 ice cubes

Directions

Blend all the ingredients.

Green Banana Smoothie

1/2 cup milk

1/2 cup vanilla yogurt

2 tsp. honey

1/4 tsp. cinnamon

2 bananas

1 cup spinach

4 - 5 ice cubes
Directions
Blend all the ingredients.

Watermelon Smoothie

2 cups watermelon
1 cup spinach
1/2 cup strawberries
1/2 cup frozen peaches
4 - 5 ice cubes
Directions
Blend all the ingredients.

Green Peanut Butter Smoothie

1 cup skim milk
3 tbsp. peanut butter
2 cups spinach
1 banana (frozen, chopped)
Directions
Blend all the ingredients.

Green Classic Strawberry Banana Smoothie

1/2 cup water
1/2 cup skim milk
1/2 cup vanilla yogurt
2 tsp. honey
1 cup mixed greens
1/2 cup strawberries
1 banana (frozen, chopped)
4 - 5 ice cubes
Directions
Blend all the ingredients.

Green Almond Dream

1 cup almond milk
3 tbs. almond butter

1 cup kale
1 cup spinach
1/4 cup blueberries
1/4 cup blackberries
4 -5 ice cubes
Directions
Blend all the ingredients.

Green Fruit and Nut Smoothie

1 cup almond milk
1/4 cup sunflower seeds
1/4 cup cashews
3 cups spinach
2 dates
1/2 cup blueberries
1 banana
4 - 5 ice cubes
Directions
Blend all the ingredients.

Minty Green Smoothie

1/2 cup apple juice
1 tbsp. ground ginger
1/4 cup mint leaves
1 cup spinach
1cup kale
1 pear
4 - 5 ice cubes
Directions
Blend all the ingredients.

Do not be afraid to play around with the recipes and tweak them. Personalize them according to your personal taste and preferences. Make them your own. As long as it is healthy and tasty, it will be a great way to start your morning with a good amount of nutrition and energy.

Samantha Michaels

CHAPTER 5- 14 GREAT SNACK GREEN SMOOTHIE RECIPES

The juicing trend isn't going anywhere anytime soon. It's long been understood that fruits and vegetables are some of the most nutrient rich sources that we, as humans, can consume. Many people have failed to find tasty ways to incorporate them into meals, especially when heat draws out the important vitamins and minerals. That's why juicing works perfectly. It gives us an opportunity to get a refreshing, and potent dose of these super foods in an easy to swallow drink.

For a long time, it was widely believed that juicing was only for detoxing and diets. In reality a zesty green drink can make an excellent snack or meal replacement that will leave you feeling revitalized and ready to take on the day. Here are fourteen recipes that do the trick.

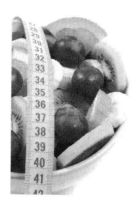

Green Powerhouse

1 Bunch Kale
½ Cucumber
4 Celery Stalks
1/3 Fennel Bulb and Stalk

1 Green Apple

1 Fuji Apple

1 Pear

½ Lemon

1 Inch Ginger

Blend all ingredients to combine.

Stomach Soother

1 Small Head of Fennel

2 Stalks Celery

1 Handful of Mint

1 Bunch Flat Leaf Parsley

½ Green Apple

2 Small Lemons

Blend all ingredients to combine.

Fennel is a surprise ingredient that's popping up more and more in the culinary world. From cold salads to creamy sauces, its bold, licorice like flavor adds a zing to many a dish. However, its uses span far outside the world of taste, in fact its health benefits are rather startling. That's why it's becoming ever present in juicing recipes.

Above all it is a helpful digestive aid. In fact, many parts of the world serve fennel seed after a meal to aid in the process. Most of the essential oils found in fennel are enhance production of gastric juices, and simultaneously reduce stomach inflammation. These components can be a cure all for an upset stomach, helping with everything from flatulence to diarrhea. Additionally the presence of Cineol and Anetol, natural expectorants, make it ideal for relief from respiratory ailments.

Immune Booster

½ Cucumber

2 Stalks Celery
Handful of Spinach
1 Apple
½ Lemon
1 Inch Ginger

Blend all ingredients to combine.

Ultracool Green Drink
8 Kiwis
3 Green Apples
1/3 Cucumber
1 Piece of Fresh Ginger
Handful of Fresh Mint

Blend all ingredients to combine.

Healthy Lungs
1 Cucumber
1 Head Romaine Lettuce
1 large Handful of Parsley
2 Meyer Lemons
1 Apple
1 Inch Ginger

Blend all ingredients to combine.

Ginger is one of those ingredients that is centuries old and is both flavorful and powerful. It is a natural anti-inflammatory and has been shown to have dramatically impressive results in persons suffering from arthritis. Most importantly it is a powerful immune booster.

Zesty Afternoon Snack
3 Apples
1 Cucumber
1 Lemon

Samantha Michaels

5 Kale Stalks

Blend all ingredients to combine.

Spinach with Pineapple and Cucumber
½ Pineapple
1 Cucumber
2 Bunches of Spinach

Blend all ingredients to combine.

Metabolism Booster
1 Cucumber
3 Stalks Celery
Handful of Fresh Mint
2 Kale Leaves
1 Peeled Lemon

Blend all ingredients to combine.

Ultragreen Wake Up
1 Pear
1 Cucumber
4 Stalks Celery
3 Sprigs Mint
4 Small Limes

Blend all ingredients to combine.

Afternoon Cooler
1 Apple
1 Pear
½ Cucumber
3 Kale Leaves
Handful Fresh Mint

Blend all ingredients to combine.

Cucumbers are full of B vitamins and electrolytes. It is ideal to reboot the body after a workout or even a rough night. They are full of dietary fiber and have a high water content making them a filling snack or the perfect complement to other nutrient rich ingredients in a green smoothie. The vegetable is also a dense source of silica, a substance whose properties are purported to improve joint health.

Stimulating Smoothie
1 Bunch Kale
Large Handful of Fresh Mint
2 Apples
1 Lemon Peeled

Blend all ingredients to combine.

Citrus Delight
4 Cups Spinach
1 Bunch Kale
2 Oranges
1 Cucumber

Blend all ingredients to combine.

Spring Green Super Shake
1 Green Apple
1 Navel Orange Peeled
1 Bunch Spinach
4 Swiss Chard Leaves
2 Kale Leaves

Blend all ingredients to combine.

Island Paradise
1 Mango
2 Handfuls of Wheatgrass
3 Handfuls Romaine Lettuce

1Cucumber

2 Pears

2 Handfuls Kale

Coconut Water

Blend all ingredients to combine.

Perhaps the most typically found ingredient in green juices, Kale is often referred to as the "Queen of Greens." The low calorie, high fiber vegetable is packed with vitamins that make every bite a potent nutritional punch. Kale has more iron per calorie than beef, a heavy dose of Vitamins K, A, and C, is filled with antioxidants and calcium and works as a high functioning anti-inflammatory. All of these properties have been shown to fight against various cancers, promote bone health, and slow neuro-degenerative disorders, like Alzheimer's.

When juicing, it's important to remember that taste is what will keep you coming back for more, day in and day out. It's hard to keep up the habit when you're downing a glass of what tastes like an undressed salad. That's why so many recipes have a sweet and citrus kick.

The good news is, most of the fruits that make these juices taste great have exciting health benefits as well. Apples are full of fiber and help keep your day running smoothly. Citrus, like limes and lemons have regenerative properties that stimulate skin cell rejuvenation for a look that's consistently young and vibrant. Coconut water is full of electrolytes, plus the taste is a tropical delight!

CHAPTER 6- 14 GREAT LUNCH GREEN SMOOTHIE RECIPES

I can't think of anything more nutritional and delicious than a green smoothie for lunch. Below are 14 recipes delicious green smoothies you could have for lunch. Hope you enjoy them.

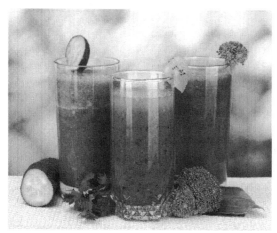

Celery Green Smoothie

1 stalk celery sliced thin

4 real ripe bananas

A handful of baby spinach

1 cup ice water or ice cubes

Directions

Add all these ingredients to the blender and puree until smooth.

Collard Green smoothie

4 oz coconut water

1 frozen banana

1 cup blueberries

1 cup seedless grapes

A handful of collard greens without the stems and stalk.

½ cup ice water or ice cubes

Directions

Add all these ingredients to the blender and puree until it is a smoothie. This one is really good. All that mixture of flavors would make a tasty lunch.

Mango Green Smoothie

1 frozen banana

1 mango sliced

2 good handfuls of baby spinach

1cup ice water

Directions

Add all these ingredients to the blender and puree until smooth

This is a very simple recipe with very few ingredients. It taste really good and will give you energy for the rest of the day.

Spicy Delicious Green Smoothie

½ cup of pure vanilla almond milk

1 banana

Dash of cinnamon

1 handful of spinach

1 tablespoon whey powder

1 cup ice

Directions

Add all these ingredients to the blender and puree until smooth.

All Purpose Green Smoothie

1 banana

1 sliced apple

1 sliced pear

1 stalk celery cut up

½ lemon

2 handfuls of spinach

1 handful romaine lettuce

Little bit of parsley

Little bit of cilantro

1 cup ice

Directions

Add all the ingredients to the blender then squeeze the lemon over it. Puree until it is smooth.

This one is delicious and perfect for lunch.

Green Tea Smoothie

1 cup green tea

1 carrot

1 banana

2 handfuls kale with the no stems or stalk

Few ice cubes

Directions

Add all the ingredients to the blender and puree until smooth. This one is a great choice for lunch.

Lemon Cucumber Green Smoothie

1 cucumber

1 pear sliced

4 celery stalks

1 peeled lemon

½ cup ice water

Directions

Add all these ingredients to the blender and puree until they are smooth. Perfect selection for lunch; this one will give you the energy you need for the rest of the afternoon.

Cashew Green Smoothie

1 cup coconut water

½ cup cashews

1 banana

2 dates

1 tablespoons flax seed

One handful of spinach

Add all the ingredients to the blender and puree until it is smooth. This one is delicious and the cashews give it something special. Great choice for lunch

Orange Green Smoothie

1 banana

5 large strawberries

½ cup peeled orange

½ cup sliced apple

Little bit of flax seed

2 handfuls of spinach

1 cup ice water

Directions

Mix all the ingredients into the blender and puree until smooth. This one is wonderful and perfect for lunch.

Fruit and Green Smoothie

1 small container plain greek yogurt

1/2cup natural protein powder

½ cup blueberries

½ cup peaches sliced

½ cup pineapple sliced

½ cup strawberries

½ cup mango sliced

1 handful of kale (remove stem and stalks)

½ cup ice water

Directions

Add all these ingredients to the blender and puree until smooth. This one is out of this world.

Ginger Green Smoothie

Small handful of parsley

1 cucumber sliced

1 peeled lemon

1 inch of ginger root

1 cup frozen apples

1 handful kale without the stems and stalks

½ cup ice water

Directions

Mix all these ingredients into the blender and puree until smooth. This one is very good. All these ingredients are wonderful together. Good choice for lunch

Melon Green Shake
½ cup black cherries pitted
1 banana
Little handful of kale cut up
½ cup blueberries
½ cup green melon
½ cup coconut water
½ cup ice cubes
Directions
Add all these ingredients to the blender and puree until it is smooth. This one is very good. All the flavors are wonderful together.

Almond Coconut Yogurt Green Smoothie
1 cup almond coconut yogurt
Bunch of cilantro
Handful of spinach
Avocado sliced
1 cup blueberries, strawberries or raspberries
1 mango sliced
½ cup coconut water
Pinch of sea salt
Ice water (as much as you need to get the thickness to your taste)
Directions
Add all the ingredients to the blender and puree until smooth. Add the water as needed. This is a delicious green smoothie with a great taste. All this mixture of flavors is a treat to drink. This recipe makes enough for 4 large smoothies.

Refreshing Green Smoothie
1 cup pineapple cut up
1 frozen banana cut up

1 mango sliced
½ cup ice water
Handful baby spinach
Directions
Add all the ingredients to the blender and puree until smooth. This one is really delicious and refreshing. This is a great choice for lunch.

These recipes are so easy and the best thing is that you can alter any ingredients to suit your personal taste. As long as you add organic fruit and some kind of vegetable greens that are healthy you can use any thing. Add ice or ice water as needed for the thickness you prefer. It does not take any time at all and no matter how busy a person they will have time to prepare these recipes.

CHAPTER 7- 14 GREAT HIGH PROTEIN GREEN SMOOTHIE RECIPES

Here are 14 awesome smoothies that will take supply the protein you need.

Cashew Blast

5-7 kernels of cashew nuts

Spinach leaves

Lemon syrup

Curd

Sugar

Directions

Half boil the spinach leaves and get rid of its raw appeal. Mix the lemon syrup and thick curd thoroughly in a bowl. Grind cashew kernels and sugar to give a coarse mixture. Put the half-boiled leaves into the curd and add the coarse cashew kernels with sugar. Finally blend a little to give a uniform texture. Enjoy this smoothie with bread toasts.

Yogurt with Cinnamon

1 ripe cucumber

1 cup oat milk

A pinch of cinnamon

Salt and coriander leaves

Probiotic yogurt

Directions

Chop the cucumber into medium sized pieces and blend all ingredients except cinnamon in a grinder. Put it into the refrigerator for a while. Just before serving, add a pinch of cinnamon and garnish with coriander leaves.

Peanuts with Mint and Honey

Peanuts without shells

1 handful mint leaves

Thick curd, honey

Ice cubes

Directions

Grind all ingredients together to form a thick uniform paste. Lastly, add the ice cubes and serve cold.

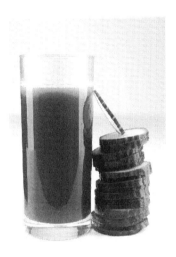

Kiwi Guava Burst

1 kiwi

1 guava, coconut water

Fresh corn kernels

Ice cubes

Directions

Chop the kiwi and guava into small pieces. Grind the corn kernels with coconut water and add the chopped fruit pieces into it. Serve with ice cubes.

Spinach Surprise

 Bread slices

Spinach leaves

Yogurt

Lemon syrup

Directions

Blend the spinach leaves in yogurt. Add bread slices and blend again to get a thick texture. Add lemon syrup to taste and serve at room temperature.

Lychee with Eggs and Honey

Egg whites

Milk

7-8 lychees

2 cucumbers

Honey

Directions

Blend the egg white thoroughly with milk and honey. Peel and chop lychees into small pieces and keep aside. Blend the cucumbers with the milk mixture. Add the lychee pieces such that they float in the smoothie. This will give flavor and taste like none other.

Almond and Banana

1 medium banana

Cubed pineapple pieces

Fresh mint leaves

Roasted almonds

Ice cubes

Directions

Slice the almonds into fine pieces and keep aside. Blend the banana, pineapple and mint leaves together with ice cubes to give slush like mixture. Garnish with slices almonds just before serving.

Lettuce with Yogurt and Orange

Organic lettuce leaves

Fresh thick yogurt

Orange pulp

Ice

Directions

Blend the yogurt with orange pulp to give a smooth pulpy texture. Half boil the lettuce and add the chopped leaves into the yogurt mixture. Blend thoroughly. Finally, add crushed ice to this mixture and serve chilled.

Pear and Banana Blast
1 organic pear
Coriander stalks
Milk
1 ripe banana
Sugar
Directions
Chop the pear into smaller pieces and keep aside. Crush the coriander stalks in milk. Add the ripe banana to milk and blend well. Add sugar to taste and add the chopped pear pieces to the smoothie. As an option, you can add mint leaves into the smoothie to enhance the taste and flavor.

Spirulina Smoothie
1 teaspoon spirulina
2-3 centimeter knob of ginger
Spinach leaves
Fruit yogurt
Hot water
Directions
Blend the spirulina with the spinach leaves together to give a thick paste. Dilute the paste with fruit yogurt according to taste and preferred texture. Boil the ginger in hot water and extract its flavor. Add the ginger extract to the mixture of spinach and spirulina. Heat the mixture till it turns lukewarm and drink the smoothie in that temperature, preferably before meals.

Fig and Walnut Smoothie
1-2 fresh figs
3 strawberries
Salt
Walnuts
Coriander leaves

Ice cubes

Milk

Directions

Add milk, strawberries, figs and coriander leaves to the milk and blend it until it turns smooth and even. Break the walnuts into smaller pieces and crush it with the required amount of salt. Add the coarse walnut crush just before you serve. Serve chilled.

Pistachios and Banana Smoothie

Pistachios

 Warm water

1 apple

1 banana

3 cucumbers

Directions

Add chopped apple pieces into warm water and crush the banana into a paste. Grate the cucumbers and add them to the banana paste. Mix the paste well and add it to the warm water containing apple pieces. Do not blend. Chop the pistachios into two and add them to the apple pulp. Now mix just the banana paste and apple pulp. Use the warm water to even out the texture. Serve warm.

Soy Smoothie

Egg whites

Soy milk

Cottage cheese

Sugar

Salt

Directions

Blend the egg whites, soy milk and cottage cheese to give a grainy texture to the smoothie. Add sugar and salt in a proportion that adds flavor to the tongue. On the smoothie, again grate some cottage cheese. For those who love cheese, this is the perfect recipe.

Cow Pea Smoothie

Samantha Michaels

Thick yogurt
Orange pulp
Cow peas
Mint leaves
Fresh onions
Protein source: egg whites, soy milk, cottage cheese.
Directions
Finely chop the onions and sauté them over a low flame. Put them aside. Half boil the cow peas so as to make them spongy and soft. Blend the yogurt, orange pulp and onions together to make a thick paste. Add the cow peas in the end. Use mint leaves to garnish it while serving. Serve chilled.

CHAPTER 8- 14 GREAT POST WORKOUT GREEN SMOOTHIE RECIPES

Banana Swiss Chard Smoothie with Lime

2 fresh or frozen bananas

3 cups Swiss chard

½ of a lime

1 cup ice

Directions

Remove stems from Swiss chard and discard.

Roughly chop Swiss chard.

Peel and segment half of a lime into small pieces. This will help when blending ingredients together.

Slice bananas into ½ inch slices.

In a blender add bananas, Swiss chard, lime and ice.

Blend on highest speed until smooth.

Spinach and Flaxseed Protein Smoothie

1 handful of spinach

1tbs tsp of flax seeds (ground)

1¼ cup coconut water

½ cup plain Greek yogurt

½ scoop vanilla protein powder

1 cup ice

Directions

Roughly chop spinach.

Add all ingredients to blender.

Blend until smooth and well mixed.

Mint Chocolate Smoothie with Spinach

1 cup milk (skim, 2 % or whole is fine)

2 handfuls of baby spinach

1 scoop chocolate protein powder

Samantha Michaels

1 scoop cocoa powder

Mint leaves (crushed)

2-3 drops peppermint extract

5 ice cubes

Directions

Crush mint leaves.

Add all ingredients into blender. Blend until smooth and creamy.

Strawberry Banana Protein Smoothie with Spinach

½ of a banana

1 cup skim milk

1 cup fresh or frozen strawberries

1 scoop of vanilla protein powder

1 handful of baby spinach

3 ice cubes

Directions

Add all ingredients into blender.

Blend until smooth.

Apple Cinnamon Smoothie with Romaine Lettuce

1 bunch of Romaine lettuce

1 banana

1 cup water

1 cup ice

½ teaspoon ground cinnamon or to taste

2 apples

Directions

Chop lettuce, banana and apples.

Add all ingredients to blender.

Blend on high until smooth.

Green Peanut Butter and Banana Smoothie

1 cup almond milk

1 tablespoon peanut butter

1 frozen banana

1 handful baby spinach

Directions
Thinly slice frozen banana.
Add all ingredients and blend on high until smooth.

Protein Pear and Kale Smoothie
1½ cups water
2 cups kale
2 ripe pears
1 frozen banana
1 scoop protein powder
¼ avocado
1 tbsp flax seed
1 cup ice
¼ cup cilantro
Directions
Roughly chop kale.
Slice frozen banana
Core pears and chop into small pieces.
Blend kale, water and herbs for on high for about one minute.
Add remaining ingredients and blend on high for about a minute or until smooth.

Mint and Pear Smoothie with Ginger
2 handfuls of kale or spinach
1 ½ cup of water
1 pear
1 piece of ginger (fresh)
Mint (to taste)
1 tsp flaxseed
Directions
Remove stems from kale.
Remove core and cut pear into pieces.
Add kale and water into blender.
Blend on high until greens are dissolved into water.
Add flaxseed and blend until broken down into mixture.
Add pear ginger and mint.

Blend until smooth.

Green Grape and Pumpkin Smoothie
2 cups green grapes (seedless)
1 pear
1 cup spinach
½ cup frozen pumpkin purée
¾ cup coconut water
Ice cubes
2 tbsp avocado
Core and chop pear.
Add all ingredients to blender. Blend on high until smooth.

Fruity Green Smoothie
6 large strawberries
½ banana
1 large orange
1/3 cup plain Greek yogurt
2 cups spinach
1 cup ice
Directions
Cut strawberries into chunks. Remove green leaves.
Slice half of banana into ½ inch pieces.
Peel and segment orange
Put all ingredients into blender.
Blend until smooth.

Simple After Workout Green Smoothie
2 cups baby spinach
½ apple
1 medium sized orange
½ lemon
1 piece fresh ginger
1 banana
2 cups water
Ice

Directions

Peel and segment orange and lemon

Peel, core and cut apple.

Slice banana.

Peel and mince ginger.

Add ingredients into blender.

Blend until smooth.

Vanilla Blackberry Green Smoothie

1 cup almond milk (unsweetened)

1 cup frozen blackberries

2 cups spinach

½ scoop vanilla protein powder

1tbsp raw pumpkin seed butter

1tsp vanilla extract

1 1/2 tbsp ground flaxseed

4 ice cubes

Directions

Place all ingredients in blender and blend until smooth.

Blueberry Celery Smoothie

2 bananas (can be fresh or frozen)

6 stalks of celery

16 oz of coconut water

2 cups frozen blueberries

Directions

Slice bananas into ½ inch slices.

Peel celery.

Add all ingredients into blender.

Blend on high for about 30 seconds or until smooth.

Mixed Berry and Banana Kale Smoothie

6 to 8 kale leaves

2 dates

4 cups frozen mixed berries

2 cups water (can also use coconut water for extra hydration)

2 bananas (fresh or frozen)
Directions
Roughly chop kale leaves.
Chop dates into small pieces.
Slice bananas into ½ inch slices.
Combine all ingredients into blender.
Blend on high until smooth and creamy.

Overall, these are 14 great post workout green smoothie recipes. Not only are they delicious but they are full of nutrients and will replenish your energy after every workout. In order to make a great green post workout smoothie all you need are some fresh greens, fruit and other nutritious ingredients such as flaxseed, protein shake powder and coconut water. Going green is both easy and delicious when it comes to smoothies. Now you don't have to spend your money on smoothies, you can follow these simple recipes and make your own.

ABOUT THE AUTHOR

Samantha Michaels is no stranger to a smoothie as she used to get smoothies from her mother all the time. Little did she know at the time that this was the method that her mother used to get her and her siblings to "eat" their vegetables!

Her mother revealed this trick to her when she gave birth to her first child and was having difficulty getting him to eat his vegetables. She thought this idea was fantastic and wondered how many other mothers knew of this trick.

She also enjoyed having smoothies as well as she was a working mother and always another go. It was a great way to get something nutritious into her system and keep her energized throughout the day.

She shared the idea with a few of her other friends and one of them encouraged her to put a guide together to inform others of how they could use smoothies for their and their families benefit.

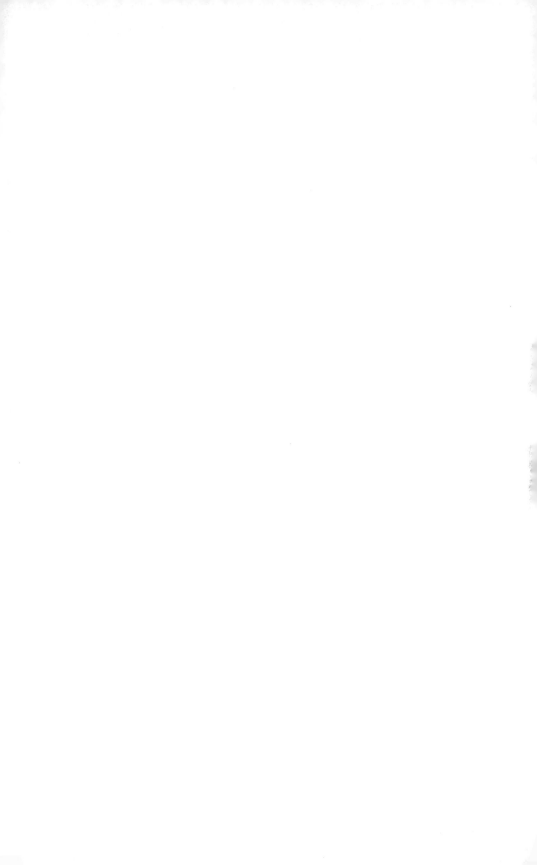

Printed in Great Britain
by Amazon